Food Addiction: Breaking the Addiction to Salt

I0440514

How to Eat Less Salt

To

Live a Healthier Life

RON KNESS

ISBN-13: 978-1535150743

ISBN-10: 1535150742

Disclaimer

All the material contained in this book is provided for educational and informational purposes only. No responsibility can be taken for any results or outcomes resulting from the use of this material.

While every attempt has been made to provide information that is both accurate and effective, the author does not assume any responsibility for the accuracy or use/misuse of this information.

Always consult your doctor before starting a fitness or diet program.

Use this information at your own risk.

Contents

Introduction

D id you know the word "salary" is derived from the word "salt"? This is because salt was so valued in ancient times that it became a form of currency, used the same then as the modern paycheck today! Interestingly, the next time you eat a salad, you should thank salt. The word "salad" is also a salt derivative, one that dates back to Roman times. This is because Romans began the practice of salting their greens thousands of years ago.

Your body needs sodium (salt) to live, so it deserves a place in your diet. Unfortunately, because of the modern day preference for fast, processed foods over veggies and fruits, you are probably getting too much salt in your diet. That over-consumption in turn can lead to multiple health issues.

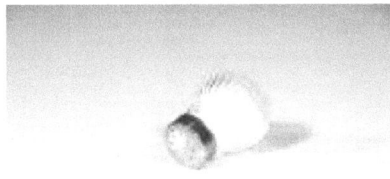

Why Too Much Salt Can Be A Bad Thing

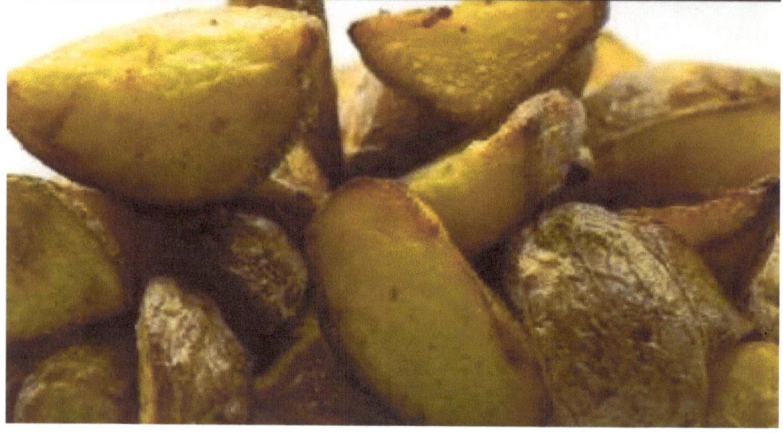

Salt is very addictive, so it takes time to train your body not to want it.

The average American consumes between 50% and 100% more salt than is recommended. Americans, and others in modern countries, take in anywhere from 3,400 to 4,500 milligrams of salt each and every day. If you eat a lot of processed and packaged foods, and your saltshaker is your friend when it comes to mealtime, the bottom line is that you are probably eating an unhealthy amount of salt.

Why is that a problem?

The United States Center for Disease Control (CDC) preaches prevention as well as treatment where disease is concerned. Research they released in 2009 shows that "70% of US adults eat 2.3 times the healthy amount" of sodium. Since then, salt consumption has risen, meaning that you are probably consuming way too much salt for your own good.

Here are just a few of the health problems linked with a high salt diet.

High blood pressure (hypertension) is the leading cause of heart attacks, heart failure, strokes and other heart diseases. Heart disease is the leading cause of disability and death in the 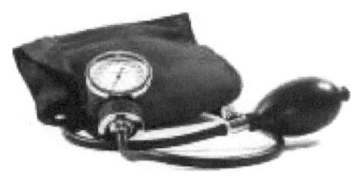 United States, the United Kingdom and other modernized nations. If heart disease was the only way that consuming too much sodium could harm you, that would be enough of a reason to cut back on your salt intake.

However, the negative effects of too much salt on the human body don't stop with heart-related problems. A high salt diet elevates your risk of contracting stomach cancer.

In the United Kingdom, 25% of the newly diagnosed stomach cancer cases each year are directly attributed to eating too much sodium.

Osteoporosis is a condition which causes your bones to be brittle, weak and thin, increasing your likelihood of broken bones. Eating too much salt causes calcium to be drawn from your bones and excreted through your urine as a waste product. High blood pressure, a salt-related health problem mentioned earlier, causes even more calcium to be removed from your bones, exacerbating the problem.

Human beings are fatter than they ever have been in human history. Salt does not directly cause you to gain weight and become overweight or obese. However, when you eat a lot of salt you are constantly thirsty. If you drink unhealthy, sweet, sugary drinks, soft drinks and energy drinks, this can lead to weight gain.

Unnecessary weight gain also come from the water retention that salt encourages. Asthma, kidney disease, kidney stones, diabetes and vascular dementia are also related to a high salt diet. Vascular dementia describes improper brain functioning that negatively affects your judgment, thinking, behavior, memory and language skills.

How Much Salt is Okay?

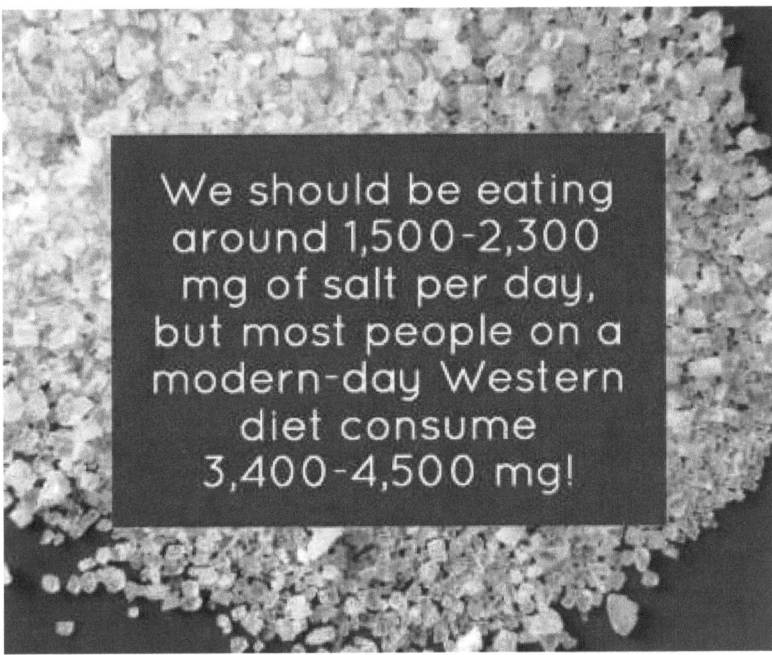

We should be eating around 1,500-2,300 mg of salt per day, but most people on a modern-day Western diet consume 3,400-4,500 mg!

In the United States, the Federal Drug Administration (FDA) has proposed guidelines in 2016 to reduce the amount of sodium in packaged food, and in restaurants. Health authorities in the United Kingdom, Canada and elsewhere are also currently (May 2016) looking into reevaluating their daily salt recommendations. What does the FDA have to do say about your recommended sodium intake?

First off, the FDA recognizes that people eating a typical Western diet consume too much sodium. This is because today's fast food society does not eat enough fresh fruits and vegetables.

The typical modern-day plate is made up of only 5% fruits and veggies. The other 95% is composed of fast foods, processed foods, bread and meat. This is simply an average, so your numbers may differ.

However, even if you eat 4 times the fruits and vegetables of the typical modern-day meal, still only 20% of your food intake is virtually sodium free. Processed foods, bread, fast foods and many meats are chock full of sodium. This is for preservation and flavor reasons. This typical diet leads to an over-consumption of sodium.

If you want a hard target, the FDA **recommends consuming no more than 2,300 mg of sodium each day.** That is roughly the equivalent of 1 teaspoon. The American Heart Association wants you to eat even less salt. They recommend the general population **should not take in more than 1,500 mg of sodium on a daily basis,** about 2/3 of a teaspoon.

Stick to those guidelines and you'll reduce your risk of contracting the dangerous health conditions mentioned above.

The 2016 proposal by the FDA to reduce salt intake includes 2 and 10-year goals. While they recommend the 2,300 mg RDA mentioned earlier, they recognize that some people are eating as much as twice that amount of sodium every day.

Their short-term goal is to educate the public so that the US average will drop to 3,000 mg per day in the next 2 years, and hopefully lowering to a safe 2,300 mg level by 2026.

You may have found it hard in the past to eat a healthy amount of sodium. You might have made heartfelt efforts to cut back on your salt intake. If you have tried and failed, the truth is, it may not be your 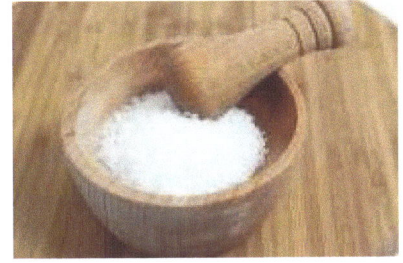 fault. You may be addicted to salt. Before you scoff at that idea, you have to understand how your brain responds to sodium.

The Salt-Brain Connection

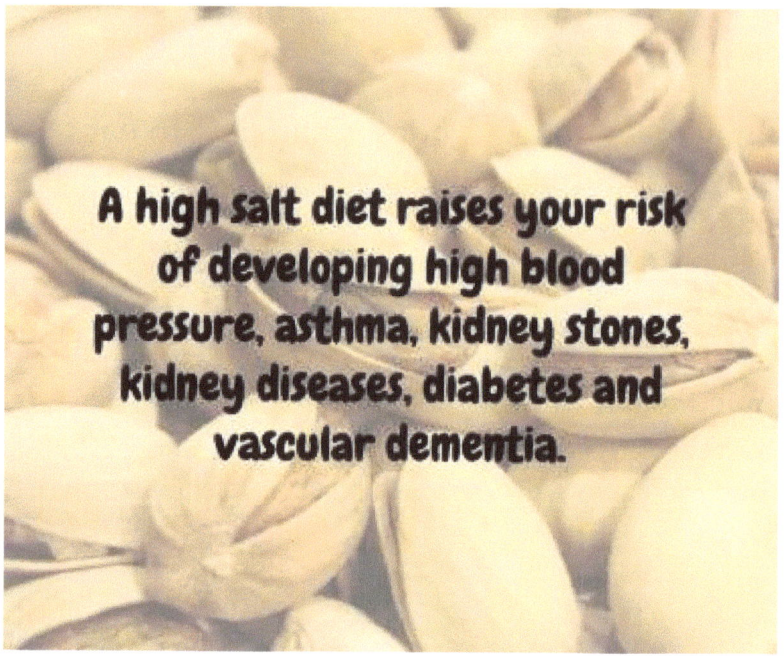

A high salt diet raises your risk of developing high blood pressure, asthma, kidney stones, kidney diseases, diabetes and vascular dementia.

Your body needs sodium for you to be healthy. So when your brain realizes that you are eating sodium, it gives you a mental "thumbs up" approval. Unfortunately, the part of your brain that responds to you putting sodium into your body also happens to be the part which controls addiction and appetite.

Scientists at the Duke University Medical Center agree with separate findings made by Melbourne, Australia researchers. Both of those studies, conducted in the early 21st century, could explain why many people have a problem eating food without sprinkling an unhealthy level of salt on it first.

Basically put, when you eat salt the pleasure center in your brain is turned on. Your appetite control weakens at the same time. This stimulates your hunger for more salt, meaning that over time, you have to eat more and more sodium to feed your growing need. The researchers mentioned above have found that this process creates a response to salt in some people that is as equally addictive as a cocaine, heroin or alcohol addiction.

Is it possible to beat such a powerful, natural process that is occurring in your brain? The answer is yes, you can overcome an unhealthy salt addiction, and in less time than you probably thought.

Beating A Salt Addiction

You can change your salty ways in as little as 21 days – the time it takes to establish a good healthy lifestyle habit (or break a bad one). Honestly, a lifetime of addictive salt consumption really can be reversed in a short period of time. Your body is such an amazing machine, and it wants to be healthy.

When you join your body and your mind in seeking healthy behaviors, you can quickly undo just about any negative habits.

Conscious efforts turn into unconscious, automatic habits in roughly 21 to 28 days.

This happens when you practice something continually, at least once a day, therefore triggering your brain's desire for order and automation. The human brain loves standard operating procedures (SOPs).

Anything that your brain can put on autopilot frees it up to spend more processing power on "one-of-a-kind" or infrequent operations and reactions.

How can you use this natural inclination to your advantage?

Start using the less salt today. Don't try to beat this powerful addiction overnight, and go cold turkey. Instead, use a little less salt in each of your meals today. Start shopping for low sodium versions of your favorite foods. Refer to the low sodium and high sodium food lists provided at the end of this report.

Slowly cut back on the number of times you eat at fast food restaurants, and the amount of processed foods you eat at home. Practice these habits, without fail, for 3 to 5 weeks. This simple, gradual, baby-step process to training your system works with any addiction, and any other time you want to trade a bad habit for good.

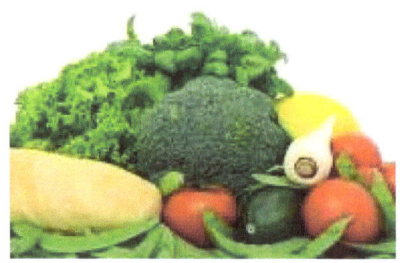

Reading Food Labels

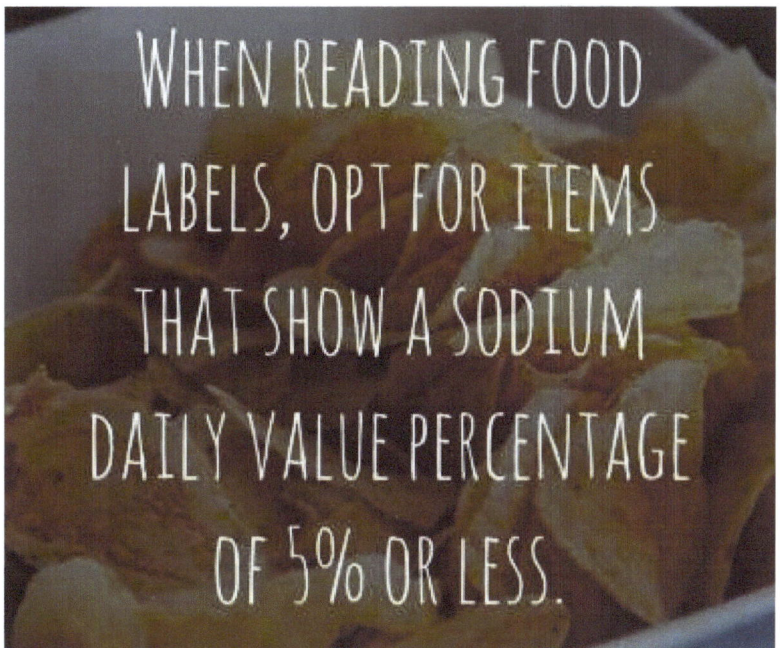

WHEN READING FOOD LABELS, OPT FOR ITEMS THAT SHOW A SODIUM DAILY VALUE PERCENTAGE OF 5% OR LESS.

One of the best ways to lower your salt intake dramatically is to choose foods with no food label! Fresh apples, bananas, kale, oranges and other non-packaged produce are as close to their natural form as you can get. This means that salt has not been added to these wonderfully healthy natural products.

With packaged food, you should always check food labels. Food labeling guidelines were made for a reason. They exist to let you know what makes up the product you are about to buy. Sodium, trans fats, saturated fats, carbohydrates and calories are all things that you should be looking for on a food label.

In the United States, sodium is usually the fourth item listed on the Nutrition Facts label. It is listed after calories, total fat and cholesterol. So, if you are looking at the nutrition label on a can of green beans, and the sodium measurement is 250 mg, is that good or bad?

Nutrition Facts

Serving Size 8 oz (227 g/8 oz)
Servings Per Container About 3

Amount Per Serving

Calories 180	Calories from Fat 60

	% Daily Value*
Total Fat 6g	10%
Saturated Fat 1g	5%
Trans Fat 0g	
Cholesterol 5mg	2%
Sodium 75mg	3%
Total Carbohydrate 26g	9%
Dietary Fiber 5g	19%
Sugars 11g	

Protein 8g

Remember that nutrition labels list how much sodium is present "per serving".

At the top of the food label, you will see "servings per container" listed. Multiply this number times the per serving sodium level, and you get an idea of how much sodium is present in the entire product.

With the canned green beans example, a common number of servings for a 14.5 ounce can is 3.5. Multiply this times the 250 mg per serving amount of sodium, and you realize that there are a total of 875 mg of salt in that entire can. If you ate that whole can of green beans, you would have consumed between 38% and 58% of your daily recommended allowance of sodium (depending on the particular recommendation you are following).

You should also note the "% Daily Value" number listed after sodium's mg amount. This tells you what percent of your daily recommended sodium allowance is contained in each serving.

For instance, if the % Daily Value is listed as 21%, that is extremely high. As a rule, look for foods that deliver 5% Daily Value (DV) scores or lower. Anything over 20% DV is extremely high. You should also look for foods labeled "low sodium," "reduced sodium," or "no salt added."

Cooking your own meals at home puts you in control of the ingredients you will be using. One way to cut back on sodium content when cooking is to start using more fresh fruits and vegetables.

Choosing "in season" produce means getting food when it is at its most delicious state. This cuts back on the amount of seasoning, including salt, you need to add.

You should also only add salt after you cook your food. This ensures you can taste the salt, which can be masked if added before or during the cooking process. You should also be reading food labels (as mentioned earlier). If you start with foods with low or no sodium, your end product will have less sodium.

Focus on ingredients you need to prepare yourself. Packaged, processed foods, as you will find out below, are often extremely high in sodium. It is much healthier for you to make a pizza from scratch at home, rather than cooking a

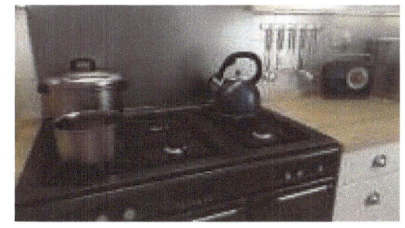

frozen pizza you picked up at the grocery store.

Opt for spices and herbs instead of salt. Garlic, Italian seasoning, rosemary, ginger, cinnamon, turmeric, black pepper, basil, chili powder and crushed red pepper flakes are just a few of the dozens of herbs and spices that deliver a no-calorie, high-flavor kick.

Make your own soups instead of heating up a canned variety. Be careful of products labeled "low-fat", as they add salt and/or sugar to replace the missing fat flavor.

Tips for Reducing Salt When Eating Out

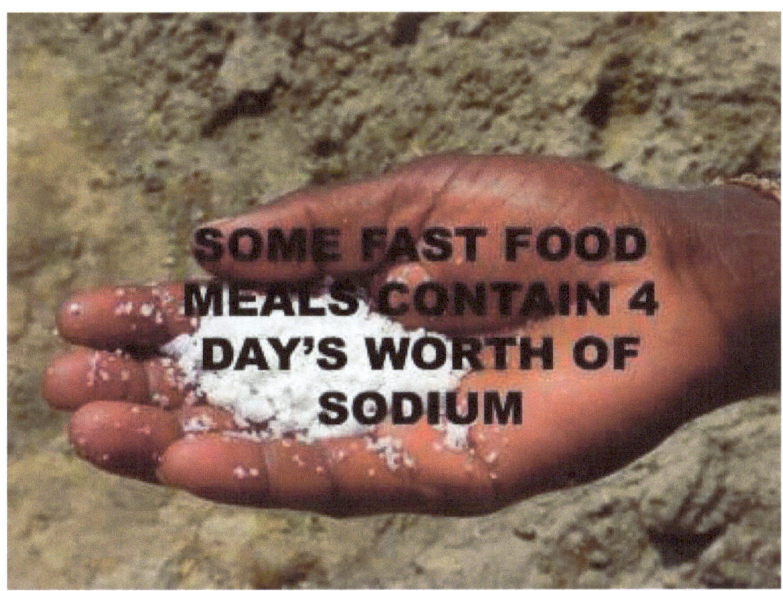

The health-oriented WebMD has revealed some startling information regarding sodium in restaurant food items. An article published on their website by Dr. Kathleen M. Zelman, MPH, RD, LD, reported the following.

> "The watchdog group Center for Science in the Public Interest found that 85 out of 102 meals at popular (US) restaurant chains contained more than a full day's worth of sodium. Some of the meals had 4 days' worth of sodium."

The proposed FDA salt reduction policy includes voluntary restriction goals for the food industry. This means that in the future, in the United States, you may be exposed to less sodium when you eat out than you are today. While that is certainly good news, you are the only person

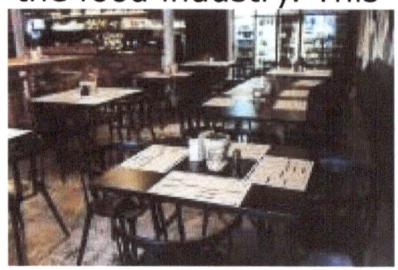

responsible for how much salt you consume.

Don't wait for someone else to help you eat healthier. There are certain steps you can take to reduce just how much salt gets into your body when you eat at restaurants, and at parties, celebrations and get-togethers. The following tips are easy to put into practice, and can help you begin today returning your salt consumption to a healthy level.

- If you're headed to a party or get-together, **prepare a dish yourself** – This is the simplest way to avoid a sodium overload. If you are attending an event or celebration that requires a covered dish, provide plenty of home-prepared low-sodium entrées and side items.

- **Avoid fast food restaurants -** McDonald's, Burger King, Taco Bell and Wendy's are examples of popular fast food destinations with extremely high levels of sodium in much of their food.

- **Order fresh fruit for dessert.**

- **Skip the "fast casual" restaurants -** These are restaurants or dining facilities which do not offer full table service, but promise to deliver a "healthier than fast food" experience. They include Panera Bread, Starbucks, Smashburger, MacAlister's Deli, Jason's Deli, Zaxby's, Chipotle, Five Guys and other similar dining destinations.

- **Bring your own –** Why not provide your own low-sodium spices and condiments?

- **Beware of Asian and Italian cooking –** Thai, Japanese and Chinese restaurants use lots of sauces. High sodium foods like soup and chicken stock are also used to prepare many of their menu items. Italian restaurants that use canned tomato products and sodium-rich cheese should be avoided as well.

- **Stick to grilled, roasted or baked foods,** and skip the casseroles.

- **Ask questions –** When you dine out, either at a friend's house or restaurant, ask a lot of questions. How else will you know exactly how much sodium is in the foods you will be eating?

- **Skip the sauce –** Sauces, even in very small quantities, are often extremely rich in sodium.

- **Choose locally owned "mom-and-pop" restaurants** – Independently owned one-of-a-kind restaurants and diners often times make food to order. This makes it easier for them to honor your no-sodium or low-sodium quests.

- **Taste your food before salting.**

Foods to Look Out For

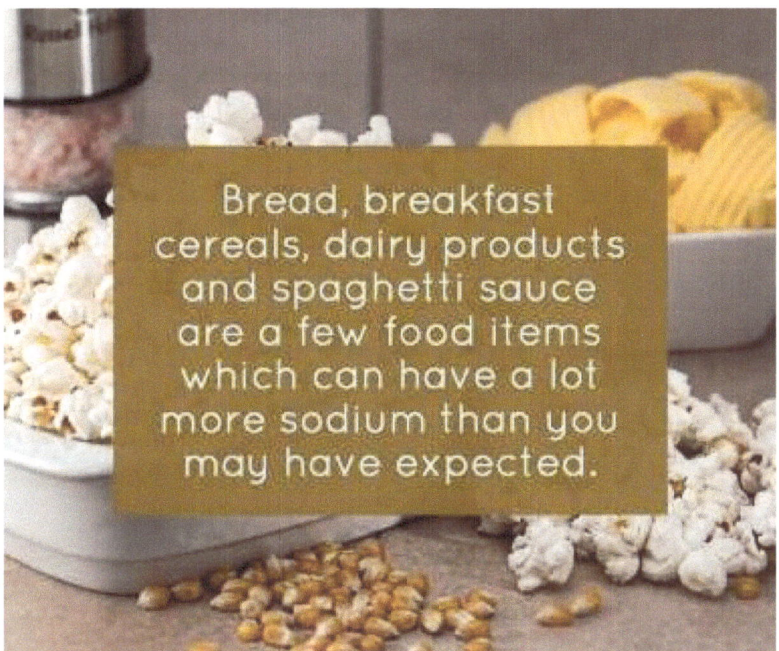

Bread, breakfast cereals, dairy products and spaghetti sauce are a few food items which can have a lot more sodium than you may have expected.

S alt can truly be a killer. That was covered earlier. You also learned how to properly read food labels, which can help you locate hidden sodium. You now know how to retrain your system, and your taste buds, to enjoy less salt. You learned how to cook with less salt, and you know how to cut back on your salt intake when you eat out.

One of the best ways to consume less salt is to understand how much salt is already in the foods that you eat.

Some foods, like bread, contain more sodium than you might imagine.

Processed foods and fast foods are notoriously high in salt as well, placed there intentionally because of the addictive properties mentioned earlier. According to Columbia University researcher Wahida Karmally, Dr. PH, RD, "**... 3/4 of the sodium in our diets comes from processed foods.**"

(If your food comes in a can, package or wrapper, it has been processed.)

Listed below are some common foods that contain higher than healthy amounts of sodium (per serving). Remember, these are just averages. If you eat any of the food items listed below, you could ingest more or less sodium.

However, these food products give you an idea of what to steer clear of so that you don't go over your recommended daily sodium allowance. (Remember to check food labels whenever available.)

- The majority of processed foods and fast foods (this is food that comes in a package, wrapper or can)
- Fried foods
- Table salt, baking soda, baking powder
- Soy sauce, teriyaki sauce, oyster sauce
- Salted fish
- Canned anchovies
- Broth cubes
- Pork bacon
- Dried beef
- Cured or deli meats like turkey, bacon, salami
- Breakfast cereals
- Canned and bottled vegetable juices
- Canned soups

- Spaghetti sauce
- Bread and tortillas
- Canned seafood
- Dairy products
- Frozen meals
- Beef jerky
- Smoked salmon
- Roquefort and Seco cheeses
- Pickles, olives, pickled eggplant, sauerkraut
- Instant soups
- Roasted and salted seeds and nuts
- Ranch and other salad dressings
- Pretzels and potato chips
- Some canned vegetables (read your nutrition labels)

Low Sodium Foods

Here are a few healthy foods which contain little or no sodium. Eat more of these, and less of the foods just listed, and you could see healthy weight loss, improved heart health, and other benefits.

- Fresh fruits and vegetables (unpackaged)
- Frozen vegetables (without added sauce)
- Dried and frozen fruit (unsweetened)
- Canned fruit (packed in water, not syrup)
- Canned vegetables (with no salt added)
- Dried beans and peas
- Pasta and rice
- Unsalted popcorn
- Unsweetened oatmeal
- Fish and shellfish
- Chicken and turkey breast (without skin)

- Lean beef and pork
- Eggs
- Fat-free or low-fat milk and yogurt
- Ketchup with no salt added
- Vinegar
- Unsalted margarine
- Natural herbs and spices
- Ginger

Conclusion

Many people don't worry about sodium in their diet unless their doctor has specifically told them to cut down on it. So they sit down to an otherwise healthy meal absent of high fat and calories and then spoil it by using an excessive amount of salt.

Even without adding sodium to your plate, your diet is probably already exceeding the normal limits of what the FDA recommends. Since most people habitually add salt to their meals, the doses they're receiving cause them to take in up to three times as much sodium as necessary.

This overdosing on salt leads to over 150,000 deaths each year, so it's vital that you shake your sodium habit and learn to infuse flavor without risking your health. One way to add flavor without the negative side effect salt delivers is to use a quick spray of lemon juice or a pinch of sugar on your foods instead. Both of these options help bring out the natural freshness and flavor of vegetables.

Garlic, dill, basil, and parsley also allow you to pull out the flavor of the food without having to rely on sodium to do the job for you. While sodium is the flavor enhancer of choice for most households, many canned, processed, and even frozen foods are already full of this ingredient.

In fact, a single fast food meal can supply more than twice your daily limit of sodium.

The biggest offenders for over-delivering on sodium are cheese, bacon, and soy sauce. Instead of using these ingredients, spice up your dish with ginger, rice vinegar, or lime juice.

Some foods mask their sodium content so that you don't even know it's in there. A Java Chip Frappuccino from Starbucks packs in 300 mg of sodium. Baked cookies, doughnuts, and bread can contain baking soda, which houses 1,259 mg of sodium *per teaspoon*.

If you want to cook some vegetables and flavor them up, instead of reaching for the salt shaker, try roasting them in an effort to caramelize their natural sugars. This brings out a rich flavor that will replace your craving for salt once your taste buds get used to it.

Make immediate choices to cut down on the excessive sodium in your diet. Too much of this ingredient can cause fluid retention, blood pressure problems, and artery damage. It can also bring an elevated risk of certain cancers and cause stomach disease, and osteoporosis. Give yourself at least 30 days to begin enjoying the natural flavors of food again and you won't miss the salt you've been adding to your diet.

Other Health Reports by This Author

If you would like to read more health reports on various topics, here is a list of CreateSpace titles and descriptions:

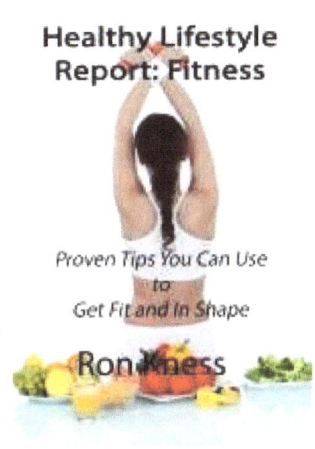

Fitness

So how much will you need to work out to feel these benefits of exercising? That all depends on your current fitness levels. The good news is that just 30 minutes of exercise a day is enough to improve your health drastically. So what are you waiting for! Let's dig deeper into the world of fitness and how it can improve your life now and into the future.

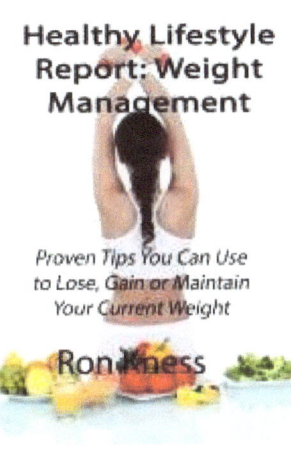

Weight Management

Losing weight in theory is easy. All you have to do is burn more calories than what you eat. If your deficit is 3,500 calories in a week, you'll lose one pound.

The problem is there are many more factors at play that can affect weight loss than just calories, such as emotions, stress, illness, hormones, menstruation, etc. So it is not easy, but with a healthy lifestyle program it is doable.

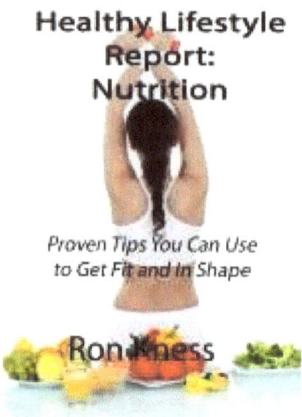

Nutrition

Nutrition is at the heart of losing weight and good health. In fact 80% of weight loss has to do with eating healthy with the other 20% about exercise. Good nutrition starts with three areas:

What you eat

How much you eat

When you eat.

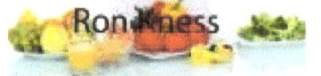

Senior Health

Retirement should be one of the best times of your life, but health issues caused by being overweight can not only limit your mobility, but cause a whole host of health problems. In this report, we discuss how to eat right, exercise and deal with some of the issues of aging.

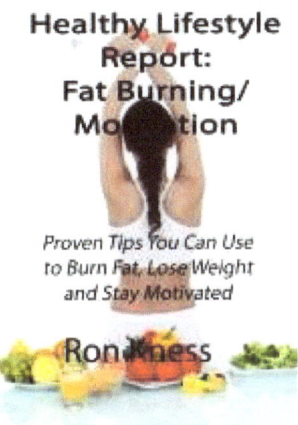

Fat Burning/Motivation

Be honest: When you look in a mirror, which bit do you hate the most? Is it those 'Love Handles' that have sprouted up?

This excess fat goes on so easy, so why does it require so much effort to make it come off again? Is it possible to burn more fat? Yes it is and we show you how in this report , along with giving you some motivation to keep going on your weight loss journey.

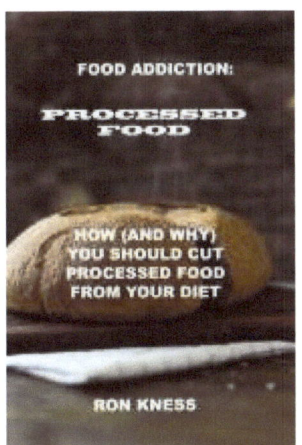

Food Addiction: Processed Food

Food addiction is one of the reasons why we as a people are so fat. But it is not all your fault.

Food manufacturers and processors add salt, sugar, dietary fat and other chemicals into the prepared and processed food we buy. Because of all the junk, our brains can't discern when we are full so we keep eating (and buying -just as they wanted) more food and the cycle continues.

But you can break that cycle and eat healthy. You just have to know what to look for - exactly what is in this report.

We'll show you what to look for on nutrition labels to tell if a food contains unhealthy ingredients along with how to prepare you own healthy food - and save both time and money by doing it.

Unhealthy eating because of food addiction is at the heart of many of our health problems of today. Don't fall prey to them because you don't know how to eat healthy. Start making the change today so you can have a healthier tomorrow.

Be sure to check back at CreateSpace at *https://www.createspace.com* frequently for new health reports. Just go to the Store and Search for "Ron Kness" (without the quotes of course) for a list of my books and reports.

About the Author

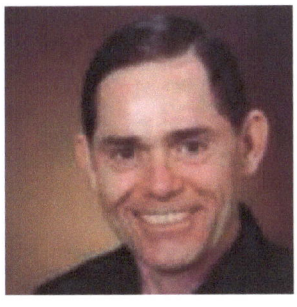I grew up in Central Minnesota, where my parents owned and operated a fishing resort. Once out of high school I tried a couple of semesters of college, only to quit halfway through the Spring term; I decided at that time that college wasn't for me.

Then I decided to follow my father's previous occupation as an auto mechanic. I graduated from a two-year of vocational training course and worked as a mechanic. While in vocational training, I decided to join the National Guard where I eventually ended up working full-time for 32 years.

So how does all of this relate to writing? In one of my leadership schools, the instructor, who was an English teacher at a juvenile detention center, presented writing to me in a whole new way - a way that started to develop my interest in working with words.

Fast forward about 40 years and I now have over 50 books listed on Amazon for Kindle and CreateSpace.

Besides my own writing, I also ghostwrite ebooks, reports, articles, blogs and do Kindle conversions for my clients on a variety of topics.

Today my wife and I live in Gold Canyon, AZ, where you'll find me happily sitting in my office typing away on my laptop as I work on my next book or ghostwriting project . . . that is if we are not traveling on a cruise ship - our new-found mode of travel.

www.ingramcontent.com/pod-product-compliance
Lightning Source LLC
Chambersburg PA
CBHW050907290526
45792CB00002B/724